Monday Night Knife & Gun Club

by L.S. Collison

Episode #4

Nurse Kit Carson's Adventures

America's New Wild West

Read 'em and weep, Senator.

Cover design by M.G. Manelis

ISBN: 978-1-7322290-3-7 (electronic)
ISBN: 978-1-7322290-4-4 (paperback)

'Funny that a dream can be catching...'

Thank you, Kevin Foster, for your inspiration.

Monday Night

Calamity

Cough cough bang! Calamity heard it, for reals. The sound woke her up. Something was chasing her. A giant bug was chasing her, Mommy and Wyatt, too. Mommy was coughing and she was shooting at the bug, but it kept on coming, the bullets did not stop it, did not even slow it down. Wide awake now, she covered her mouth to hold back a cough. Mommy! She didn't dare say it out loud. Mommy's at work taking care of sick people, maybe saving their lives, so don't be a baby, Cal, it was only a dream, that's what Wyatt would say. She reached for Dolly, her rag doll, couldn't find her in the tangle of covers. Where was Dolly? Wyatt and Mike, playing in the living room; in her mind's eye she could see their thumbs on the controllers, the cowboys moving across the screen, chasing the bad guys. "Got you, you dirty bastard!" Calamity curled up in a ball beneath the blankets. Keep still. Don't make a sound. But what if that's where the bugs can get you—in your dreams? She hoped Mommy would be OK.

Tonto

Tim Rhodes clipped his I.D. badge onto the pocket of his scrubs.

Tonto RN
www.WellmartEmergency.com
Like us on Facebook
Follow us on Twitter and Instagram
Healthcare the American Way

There was a barcode to scan for charging meds, dressings, and other supplies. In the bottom right hand corner, his photo. Clean-shaven, hair pulled back in a long braid, a braid once black, now iron gray. Stoic expression.

The whole Emergency staff went by aliases, avatars that represented their personae. Tim had chosen a culturally appropriated, demeaning Hollywood stereotype, embracing it, rebranding it, owning it entirely. The aliases also protected their real names from the public, from patients and vengeful families who might seek retribution or retaliation for some imagined medical misstep. And now the alias also protected him against the Corporate outlaws. More than ever, he was glad for the anonymity.

After scanning his barcode to clock in, Tim took report from the off-going nurse, whose soiled duster and bandanna now lay in a heap in the corner.

"Shit keeps changing", she said, stripping off her gloves. "New orders coming down from Corporate by the hour about who gets treated and how." One thing didn't change, and that was the need for hands-on care. Care and personal protective equipment, which was in short supply.

Tim Rhodes didn't work for the Wellmart Corporation, he worked for the per diem nursing agency. As such, he had the freedom of choosing where and when he worked, and got paid by the hour—almost twice what Wellmart's nurses made—but per diem nurses had no benefits, such as pension, paid vacation, health insurance. Sometimes the work dried up because the hospitals all staffed according to census, and if they could do without a nurse, the corporate bean counters made damn sure they did. But lately there had been plenty of work. Wellmart would have hired him on as one of theirs, but Rhodes didn't want to give up his freedom.

That day, he had worked with the Vigilante Volunteers, making home visits, taking isolated ranch folk coffee and donuts, checking their temperatures and their blood pressures, helping them deliver hay to the cattle still up in the north forty. The flu season had been a bad one. Pneumonia was a lone gunman, picking off the old and the infirm. That metaphor was appropriate for High Plains, where nearly everybody owned a firearm to protect themselves against renegade Indians, outlaws, and crazy in-laws.

In the packed waiting room the poor, tired, huddled masses sat in hard plastic chairs, like third graders waiting for the bell to ring. If they only knew the magic words, Tonto thought. 'Chest pain' or 'Difficulty breathing,' would get you seen quicker. Or if you said nothing because you were unconscious, then you didn't have to wait but were whisked through the double doors to the Treatment Area – Authorized Personnel. And, of course, if you came in by ambulance, you got the red-carpet treatment. But a ride in the lifesaving limo, that came with a hefty price. Just last night Sheriff Bully Ratzer had come in by ambulance. He went directly to ICU, he did not pass GO, he did not have to pay $200 out-of-pocket. Sheriff was on the gold-plated health insurance plan; the same one the legislators were on.

Ratzer had himself a bad case of the grippe. The grippe and psychiatric emergencies, they were keeping the nurses busy that spring. Coughers and moon-howlers, they came in droves. The psych cases, the worst ones, were put in the solitary cells at the end of the hall until the psych evaluator on call made it in. Meanwhile, the nurses kept an eye on them, the nurses and the guards. Few ER docs bothered to lay hands on the psych cases. To the compartmentalized Western medicine way of thinking, the head is separate from the body. Insurance companies denied pretty much any claim that originated north of the neckline. Hell, everybody's mind is fucked up to some degree. And so, they denied most psychiatric claims; they had to, or they'd be unable to make a profit. Profit, private enterprise, that was the American way. One by one the mental institutions closed, state hospitals shrank by half, and the poor crazies hit the streets with nowhere else to go. Except the emergency department, we take all comers.

Rhodes had been in the healthcare business long enough to know he wasn't going to change how the system operated. Sometimes a cup of kindness is the best medicine. But at Wellmart the nurses were supposed to charge for it; there was a box on the charge sheet they were required to mark if they administered kindness, empathy, or gave a listening ear.

A little after midnight, Tonto managed to break away for a five-minute weather check out on the ambulance ramp. He noticed a change in the wind direction and a halo around the waxing moon. Spring storm was brewing. Cupping his hands against the wind, he lit a cigarette. Heard the deep rumble of a Harley approaching. *Cough cough bang!* But that wasn't a Harley hiccup; Tonto's ear was keen. That bang was a gunshot. He watched as an Indian Chief Dark Horse, a real beauty, like the one Wild Bill used to ride, pulled into the Emergency parking lot, then fell over. Dropping his half-smoked cigarette, he pulled out his phone and punched in a code red before sprinting across the asphalt to where the victim lay, beside his trusty ride.

It *was* Wild Bill. Now, who would want to shoot that old man? One of the rival biker gangs would likely be blamed for the sake of convenience, but Tonto knew better. There's no mistaking the sound of a thirty-caliber Springfield. Not exactly the sort of weapon the motorcycle gangs carried. Pressure on the artery, warm blood still pumping. Bill gasped and gurgled, grabbed Tonto's sleeve and tried to tell him something.

Once they had Wild Bill inside, the team coded him for forty-eight minutes, but it was no use, the old man was a goner. If the bullet hadn't got him, would the grippe have done him in? Or would he have lived many more moons until the chronic obstructive pulmonary disease killed him? Wild Bill was a heavy smoker, but who's to say? You can extend life so long but, in the end, something gets you. The heart fails, the kidneys, or the lungs turn to sponge. The last few weeks of April had seen more deaths than High Plains was accustomed to handling; it was like a big snow-dump of deaths. The old man's friend, that's what they used to call pneumonia. When your life's bills were all mounting, coming due, and it was time to pay the reaper, pneumonia was the one that raised the red flag to the bill collector in black, the guy with the scythe. Pneumonia isn't one specific disease, it's a catchall term for an infectious process in the lungs. It can be viral or bacterial, it can be caused by inhaling something toxic or by inhaling a bit of food—aspiration pneumonia. This grippe caused pneumonia, it caused the body's immune system to go to war against the little bastards, and sometimes major organs got killed in the crossfire. Collateral damage. 1918 had been a bad year for the grippe, and it had been a bad year for the guys in the trenches shooting at each other across no man's land. Grippe killed more than the war. A similar bug hit us this year. Come spring, it seems to take one last stand, Custer's last stand, determined to go out in a blaze of glory, like a deranged shooter, taking as many with it as it can. Then the snow melts, summer blooms hot and dry, and everybody forgets about the grippe. Until the next bad one hits.

Kit Carson

Monday, my night off. My night to work undercover for the Vigilantes. I showed up at Wellmart in a city slicker suit, pulling a briefcase on wheels, like a pharmaceutical rep. Inside the briefcase, my costume. Thinking, I like the way my spike heels sound, the confident click they make on the linoleum floor. Excited for the card game up in the executive suite. The bigwigs meet up there every Monday night to gamble. Wells Fargo is the House, and they provide a banker to deal cards and handle the accounts. Tonight, Doc Halliday is dealing the cards, though the bigwigs don't know it. They don't know her—she's just an ER doc—and they sure as hell don't know me. They don't know any of us, even though we work right under their noses, on the ground floor beneath them.

On my way in, I saw Olinger's van at the service entrance. Word was, the bodies had been stacking up—in the hospital's cold storage, in the city morgue, in the funeral parlors up and down the Front Range. Crematoriums running day and night, and now that spring thaw had set in, graves were being dug once again.

They say this bug is different and maybe it is. If I seem jaded or blasé, it's just because I've seen a lot of people die from a lot of different causes. And it's never pretty, it's never peaceful, and it's never without collateral damage. No one ever goes gently into that good night, not that I've seen.

*

Tonight, I'm not a nurse, I'm a cocktail waitress for healthcare justice. I'll smile sweet as honey as I lean over the table to hear their order, my cleavage inches from their nose. They don't know the drinks I'll be giving them will be doctored up with MDMA, to help them open up, share their feelings, spill some secrets, show a little compassion, for a change. Maybe see beyond the bottom line.

Until tonight, I'd been keeping my head down, trying to keep food on my table, gas in my Wagon, and the rent paid. Putting in a lot of hours. Nurses are always in demand, but the bean counters don't want to pay for us. The fewer you have to pay, the better. When there's an industrial accident, a train wreck, a mass shooting, or something like that, then you call in the guns for hire—the per diem nurses—like me and Tonto.

A lot had changed in my life, the past few months; the winter had been a hard one. First, the hospital shooting that killed my best friend and shut down the last nonprofit hospital in the West. Then, the whole Bully Ratzer bullshit went down. Now, the Wether sisters were reunited and working at the casino up in Wind River under new aliases—and under the protection of the Eastern Shoshone and the Northern Arapaho—and the illegals who were living in the back of my truck have moved into my house, but that turned out to be a good thing. Wyatt and Mike are best friends, and the men have jobs, they chip in on the rent. Abuela looks after the kids when I'm at work or volunteering for the Vigilantes, and I come home every day to hot coffee, homemade tortillas, and a pot of green chili on the stove. I've learned to appreciate what's important in life, but there's something missing, something vital, I don't know what.

*

I stepped off the elevator. Wow. So this was where the gods of healthcare lived. Abstract mural on the wall looked like Picasso's Guernica. A tree growing, a real fucking ficus, reaching almost to the skylights. Night watchman at the reception desk, enjoying a cup of coffee. I smiled and held up the fake badge hanging from a lanyard around my neck. Must've looked the part because he smiled back and buzzed me into the executive suite. The double doors opened. I tried not to gawk. Man, this place is tits.

Spied the bar off to the left and ducked in. Shane, dressed smartly in slim black pants and a crisp white shirt, black garters around his sleeves, was playing the role of bartender. In real life, Shane's a nurse anesthetist.

"Where can I change my duds?"

He jerked his thumb over his shoulder, toward a restroom for the staff. I slipped in, opened my briefcase and stripped down, donning the slinky cocktail dress I'd been given to wear. Shook my hair free from the bun, arranging it over my bare shoulders. Then washed my hands in the sink, lathering up with lily-of-the-valley scented soap, taking care to clean under each nail, clipped short, filed smooth, and unvarnished. My hands were not my best feature, but they were clean hands and they were competent.

Shane whistled approvingly when I came out. He was pouring gin into a cocktail shaker.

"Give it to me straight, barkeep. Does this dress make my butt look big?"

"You say that like it's a bad thing."

"Fuck you, Shane." I smiled winsomely. Nothing like a little banter with your colleagues to make the shift bearable.

"How about giving me report? What's the low-down on our patients tonight?" From out in the next room, the conversation grew louder as more players arrived. I had come in cold on this gig and I needed some background info.

"High rollers, every one. See that guy in the white Stetson? That's J.R. Ellsworth, former CEO of Alamo Insurance, headquartered in Dallas. Now he advises the POTUS." J.R.'s diamond bolero sparkled under the track lighting. "Old oil money there", Shane added.

"Next to him, you got Slim Jim Horner, former prosecutor and now territory legislator—eager to make his mark in the political rodeo." Horner, I knew, came from a long line of Esquires and Honorables who had all held political offices of one sort or another.

"On his left there's Billy Palmer Jackson. Looks unpretentious, but don't be fooled—he's a real swingin' dick. Made a fortune in railroads and other investments. I don't know how he figures into this game, but you know what they say?"

"Say about what?"

Shane gave me a patronizing smile. "Follow the money, darlin'. You gotta be rich to be invited to play in this game. Rich and powerful. Now, sitting next to Mr. Jackson is Doctor Hook, CEO of the pharmaceutical company that holds the primary drug concession for Wellmart. Word is, he wants Alamo's contract, but he's up against Johnson & Johnson, and that's Johnson, Jr. next to him, sucking on a platinum toothpick."

I made a mental snapshot of each player and memorized their name, a little trick I had learned taking care of patients. "Whoa, who's the dame?"

"That's Lollie Lovit. I don't know what she does, a hooker or a lobbyist, I'm guessing. Keep your eye on her. She's probably a spotter for one of the big players. And, next to her, that's Little Jim Little, the Lieutenant Governor, and lastly, sitting at the head of the table and licking that big Cubano, that is Big Dick Beamis. Wellmart's head honcho, himself."

"He's shorter than I would've thought."

The top of the CEO's bald head shone pink under the overhead lights. Big Dick Beamis signed our paychecks. Well, not mine because I was a hired gun, I worked for the per diem agency and had no particular loyalty to anyone, except my patients. I collected my earnings, cash on the barrel, the morning after every shift. It was risky business, but I could not find it in myself to commit to Wellmart exclusively.

"So, who are we pulling for, Shane? What's at stake here?" I didn't know much about poker or the business part of healthcare. Hell, all I knew was how to take care of patients, how to carry out doctors' medical orders, how to help people feel better. I knew the ABCs of saving lives, but I didn't have a clue as to how to make a profit from doing so.

"Beamis is a real sumbitch," Shane said. "But he's our sumbitch." He opened a capsule and dropped the powder into a cocktail shaker full of Beefeater. "Molly here should loosen him up. Maybe make him feel a little compassion." He added another capsule, followed by a generous splash of vermouth and a scoop of ice cubes. Then, with a satisfied smile, he put the lid on and shook it lewdly in front of him, just below the level of his belt.

I gave him an eye roll. "You're disgusting."

"What? You want yours stirred?"

"Yeah." I grinned back and held up my freshly washed middle finger, making a slow circle. "Like that."

Shane poured the mixture into chilled martini glasses, added a spear of olives to each one, and placed them on a tray. "Now, git to work, cowgirl." He winked. "And don't forget your mask."

Doc Halliday

Tonto intercepted him as soon as he came through the door.

"This way," Tonto said, leading the well-dressed young man to one of the psychiatric holding rooms at the end of the hall. It was the card dealer from the house bank, Wells Fargo. He carried a briefcase with the outline of a stagecoach drawn by three horses embossed into the rich brown leather.

"But I'm not here for treatment," the man insisted. "I'm here on business. Important business."

"Standard procedure and recommended precaution," Tonto said, in a quiet but firm voice, a voice that could calm a rattling snake and convince it to slither away. "Just a routine temperature scan." The banker complied, and Ruth Halliday followed them into the room.

"Have you been out of the territory recently? Been exposed to anyone with the grippe? Exhibiting flu-like symptoms?" Tonto ran a digital thermometer across the banker's forehead.

"None of this is necessary, I assure you. The boss is expecting me upstairs."

Tonto pressed his lips together. Showed the reading to Halliday. She cocked an eyebrow with exaggerated drama, said, "Mister, I'm afraid your body temperature is abnormal. You'll need to strip down to your skivvies; we have to collect a specimen. A stool sample." That wasn't quite true; she needed his costume for a few hours. Not to mention they had run out of grippe testing kits hours ago.

"But I feel fine,"

"That's what they all say, at first. But we can't take any chances. I'll step outside, the nurse here will assist you. Oh, and I'll need to decontaminate your briefcase."

"But—"

"Standard procedure. Don't worry, you'll get it back."

Halliday left Tonto to attend to the Wells Fargo employee. The plan was to keep him locked up in the psychiatric isolation room until the card game was over. Well, at least he'd be safe in there.

*

They were running out of medical supplies, out here on the frontier. Good citizens were sewing masks from fabric scraps, God bless them, and it helped slow down the onslaught. One bug, one single virus, a packet of genes, can't kill you but an army of them can. Ruth was philosophical when it came to death. For her, life and death was a game. Death for the individual is a given, the House always wins, but when and how you die, now that's the interesting part. In some games, you can buy time, but at what price? Medicine is a numbers game, dodging stats and likely outcomes, outsmarting standard deviations, becoming an outlier on the right side of the curve. You know your odds, but still you take your chances, you play the hand you've been dealt. It's the playing that matters. There is no winning, there is only the playing. Life is a card game and death is the lone gunman who comes to collect.

Just that evening, she had seen him in the parking lot, three, maybe four, cars away. A tall figure, dressed in a long black duster and carrying a bolt action rifle. The old pit boss himself. And then he was gone—ducked down between the cars or vanished into thin air. He had let himself be seen on purpose, and Ruth Halliday was glad for the reminder. Seeing him close at hand always made her feel more alive.

Now dressed in the dealer's confiscated clothes, she felt a rush of excitement, the very act of disguise, an aphrodisiac. Crisp white linen shirt, black sleeve garters, silk bowtie, and a richly brocaded vest. Close-cropped hair greased smooth, and a paste-on 'stache under her black silk bandanna. Inside the Wells

Fargo briefcase, her own deck of cards. Halliday was a tough old buffalo soldier, a

medic in the wars before she became an Emergency Medicine physician. According

to some, the best practitioner in High Plains, before Insurance companies took

control. But the doctor's real passion was Blackjack. Blackjack and cosplay.

*

The corporate den was abuzz with conversation when she entered, using the

dealer's access badge. The old military training came back as she automatically

appraised the room in a shrewd sweeping glance, sizing up the players, making a

mental map of the space, ingress and egress, identifying possible hiding places. She

saw Kit, their eyes met briefly, casually, as the nurse flirted with the Suits,

offering them drinks, doing the form-fitting, low-cut cocktail waitress outfit

justice. They were used to working together in the ER, digging out bullets,

impactions, treating-and-streeting 'em or sending them to the floor. Working with

a good nurse was like dancing with a good partner, no convo needed. Halliday had

handpicked Kit as her protégé, saw her potential as a partner. With a little

training, that one would be an excellent card player. Like the best nurses, Carson

was a keen observer of detail with a sixth sense for subclinical symptoms. She was

new to cards, she didn't know all the rules and ramifications, but that nurse definitely had the instincts. The two of them, working a casino together, now that was pleasurable to think about. But first, to get through this night with some sort of advantage for the Vigilantes and the people of High Plains.

She stepped into the center of the gaming table with the confidence of stepping up to the bedside of a patient in full cardiac arrest. Alert, scrubbed, gloved, and masked. Eight players already seated in the oversized, overstuffed, leather chairs; on their phones, placing other wagers, in other games, countless deals going on all over the West. No masks or gloves for them. Let the little people halt the spread of grippe, the crème of High Plains couldn't be bothered. She cleared her throat, the sign for them to finish their transactions. Waited until they pocketed their phones, knowing she had 'em where she wanted 'em. Having researched their backgrounds thoroughly, she knew their salaries and their CVs, their medical histories, she knew who was premenstrual, perimenopausal, and who had erectile dysfunction. She knew what was at stake at this table tonight—the access to healthcare in High Plains. Picking up a deck in her dexterous hands— hands skilled at palpating, percussing, suturing, and sleight of hand—she shuffled the deck and went to work. Read 'em and weep.

Throwing a card game was not a sure thing. Most of the players, Halliday noticed, were playing dry and sober; their doctored drinks sat untouched in front of them, the ice melting. Lollie Lovit was a spotter; she gave herself away with her unnecessary movements, touching her ear, twirling her hair. These Monday night card games were more than good old boy camaraderie, way more. It wouldn't devolve into a corporate rave, which would have been easier to take advantage of, but Ruth Halliday, that old ace in the hole, knew more than one way to manipulate a game. She had her eye on a stockpile of valuable medical equipment and PPE needed right here in High Plains. If Big Dick Beamis played his cards right, those supplies would be his to control.

Kit

Another hand played, and if I understood it right, Wellmart's health insurance just changed to Alamo. Whether this was good or bad I couldn't say, but probably bad. There hadn't been an increase in nurses' benefits since the year the unions were run out of town. Things weren't going according to plan. The players weren't drinking anything but bottled water, the good stuff, from Italy and France. The martinis laced with molly sat untouched on the table, and instead of loosening up and growing more empathetic and loving, the players were becoming more withdrawn, getting harder to read. I was trying to learn all I could—about the game, about the stakes, about the personalities of these high rollers—by watching their plays, their body language, and reading their faces.

Big Dick started sweating profusely. He was trying hard to maintain his poker face, a face darkening from pink to purple. He looked like he could use some more water, so I brought him a fresh bottle, opened it there at the table. But something was wrong. What was it? He seemed frozen, yet there was panic in his eyes. Was he choking?

"Can I get you something else, Mr. Beamis? Mr. Beamis, are you OK?" Oh shit, oh hell, he was definitely not OK. "Can you speak? Are you choking?"

Halliday shot me a reprimanding scowl; it was out of line to talk to the players. If they wanted something, they would signal me. But I didn't care about poker etiquette; I was trying to save a life. I bent down, put my hand on his chest, felt it rise and fall. Felt his breath hot on my face. Not choking, his airway was patent. "Mr. Beamis, can you smile? Give me a smile now, will you?" I was all up in his face now, assessing his expression, looking for symmetry. This was no poker face, this was a half-paralyzed face. "Stick your tongue out, let's see some tongue." But though the left side of his face twitched, he could not do it.

The other players stared mutely, shocked at my intrusion. For a moment there was no other sound in the room but the icemaker in the bar, rattling with a new delivery of cubes. Then Halliday's stern voice, reprimanding me for interrupting the game. She was a doctor, did she not see this man was stroking out? The cards in his right hand fell to the floor. I saw a jack and a queen of diamonds face up on the hardwood. Still, the others maintained their poker faces. Did they not see? Or were they too scared to react?

"Squeeze my hands, Mr. Beamis. Squeeze as hard as you can." His left hand squeezed mine, but his right hand was lifeless. Reached for my phone, but dammit, there wasn't a pocket to be had in this ridiculously tight dress. Remembered I left my phone on the bar. "Somebody call Emergency," I said. But no one moved. "Shane!" I looked toward the adjoining room, saw him sitting at the bar chowing down on Chinese take-out, his earbuds in. I hurried over, grabbed my phone and called the Emergency Department my own damn self.

"Kate, is that you? This is Kit Carson. Send a team up to the corporate suite, asap. I've got a middle-aged white male with an acute onset of right-sided hemiparesis. The victim is conscious, but unable to speak. Stroke protocol. Call EKG, radiology, pharmacy."

"Corporate suite? Where the hell is that?"

"Five floors above you. Use your tracking device. I'll leave my phone on."

Beamis needed intravenous access and tPA to dissolve the clot. He needed blood pressure intervention and continuous monitoring; he needed an anticonvulsant. He needed a CT scan, or better yet, an MRI. Halliday knew it, Shane knew it. Was I the only one who saw what was happening? Were my colleagues too much into their alter-egos to recognize and respond appropriately? I stood by the stricken man, talking to him, my hand on his shoulder, reassuring him, and in three minutes flat the ER team had come up and rolled him away, but there was no making up for the fact that Wellmart's CEO had folded, and those stockpiled supplies we needed were not in his possession.

"Is he gonna make it?" Lollie Lovit asked, the only one who said anything. The other players looked down at their hands, not wanting to show any emotion, not while the game was in play. After all, Beamis's misfortune was none of their own. Halliday finished the round, distributed the chits, then the players got up and left. I wondered if anyone had called his wife.

Shane collected all the spiked martinis, pouring them into a gallon jug. "Can't let this stuff go to waste. Call your friends, Kit, we'll make our own little party."

I smiled and shook my head no. "Sorry, Shane. All I want is to change out of this sleazy dress and go home to my kids." Calamity had texted me about a bad dream she had. She needed her mother and I needed a good night's sleep.

But a good night's sleep was not in the cards for me. We had to get our hands on those medical supplies before they were all loaded onto Billy Jackson Palmer's freight train and hauled away.

"Kit, we need you and your wagon," Halliday said. "Meet Tonto downstairs and get going."

Tonto

Meanwhile, down in the Emergency Department, Tim Rhodes had given the Wells Fargo dealer a thorough assessment, holding him until the card game was over, performing a traditional Arapahoe prayer dance for his benefit before releasing the bewildered hostage with complimentary samples of antihistamine.

The man called Tonto felt his practice to be a pastiche of traditions and beliefs. He was a man of science, practiced modern medicine, yet he smoked tobacco on occasion, and marijuana to relax; he burned sage to purify the air, he fasted and ingested peyote for visions of clarity. The man called Tonto had built his own sweat lodge, and he sang Arapaho prayers, yet he had seen firsthand the value of third generation antibiotics, genetic testing and computerized tomography scans. He also knew there were no certain cures for any disease; a man's will to live or his wish to die could not be discounted. The man called Tonto was a white man's nurse and an Arapaho healer. He was a medicine man.

The older he got the more he felt an affinity for the old ways. He belonged to a time when his people hunted elk and bison with bow and arrow, ate the meat, the organs, used the bone and horn for tools, wrapped themselves in the hide. Animals and plants were sacred because they were alive, they sustained life, they made life possible. On the other hand, he had never once ridden a flesh-and-blood horse; but he was at one with his two-wheeled steel horse. Unlike most people of High Plains, he did not carry a gun. Yet he had killed a man with his bow and arrow. He had killed protecting others not of his tribe.

*

In anticipation of the raid on the Fort, Tonto called on his brothers, the Arapahoes and the Cheyennes, and the Old White Guys on Wheels, those bikers who collected toys for kids at Christmas and held summer rides to raise money for warriors wounded in battle. They would do it, they would all unite for a just cause, healthcare for all.

Even while the game was going on five stories above him, Tonto had done his research on the internet, in the palm of his hand. The Fort was being used as a supply depot again, just as it once had been back in the 1860's when the U.S.

government stockpiled annuities for the Indians there. The annuities—grain and other food, tools, hardware—were given in accordance to the Treaty of Fort Wise, a dubious agreement which reduced the size of the reservation the Cheyenne and Arapaho had been granted under the previous Treaty of Fort Laramie, which had been broken by the whites when gold was discovered in Colorado.

A little recon in the field by the Cheyenne named Lone Tree had determined that the supplies were already loaded into a shipping container and waiting for pick-up in the parking lot. There would be security to deal with—a locked gate, security lights, cameras, silent alarms. The trick was to get in and out quick. Tonto assigned three of his brothers to help him load. Kit would stay behind the wheel, the wagon in the get-away position.

Kit

Riding shotgun beside me, Tonto, his cell phone on speaker. He was coordinating with the bikers. We were about ten minutes out. According to Plan A, we'd load up my wagon, and then we'd be outta there in a hurry. Get in, get out, and nobody gets hurt. We hoped to have the element of surprise working for us. Tonto and me, we made quite a team, and I was proud the Vigilantes chose me to accompany him. Did Halliday know what a good team we were? Or maybe it was just my wagon they needed. I didn't care. With Tonto riding shotgun, I could've robbed a bank. Me and

Tonto, Belle Starr and Jesse James. Come summer, when all of this was past, I was

looking forward to holing up somewhere with Tonto, just the two of us, for a long

weekend together.

A pair of bolt cutters severed the chain that held the gate closed. The bikers

entered and formed a circle around the block of containers in the lot, waiting to be

picked up. One of the bikers cut the lock on one of the doors, someone shined a

flashlight inside. What the hell—coffins? We went to the next container, same

thing. Every container stacked high with them. Instead of masks, gloves, and paper

gowns, we've got caskets. Instead of lifesaving gear and equipment, we've got

fucking pine boxes.

"Look at this," Tonto said, shining the flashlight down at our feet. Fresh tire

tracks in the spring mud and a large rectangle of dry ground where another

container had been.

Our lifesaving supplies had been picked up before we got there and were

probably headed for the train depot. With a war cry, Tonto alerted his riders who

roared off to intercept them.

*

30

It hit me like an iron horse. The crushing fatigue, the fire in my joints, burning eyes, the aching in my head. Shivering, I leaned against the hood of my wagon, warm from the ride, absorbing its heat.

"Don't come too close," I warned. "Keep your distance. I've been hit."

"You've been shot?"

"No, it's the grippe, the bug, I've got it. I feel like hell."

"If you've got it, I've already been exposed," Tonto said. "Give me the keys. I'll drive us out of here."

He opened the door, he helped me into the passenger seat where I collapsed, like a marionette whose strings have been cut. Just to breathe was a supreme effort. One at a time, like climbing a mountain. Tonto at the wheel, his duster over me, a faint smell of buffalo hide, sage, and cigarette smoke, the motion of the wagon vibrating my bones, my dry and thirsty bones. Where are we going? I don't care, just keep moving, keep moving, my throat's burned dry and my soul does cry for water. Cool, clear water. Sing that song for me, would you?

Outside the window, drawing up beside us in the next lane, a white hearse, pale in the starlight. I couldn't see the driver through the tinted window, but I knew he was coming for me. The lone gunman, putting down victims one by one. Was it murder? Justifiable homicide? Or was it mercy killing? They put down dogs, don't they? Our beloved four-legged friends. But I can't die. I've got responsibilities. Who will raise my children? Long minutes passed, or was it hours, maybe days, and it occurred to me that they were already grown, Wyatt and Calamity Jane, grown and long gone, and I had missed it. But maybe it wasn't too late. Tonto was still driving, he would protect me, he was both warrior and medicine man. We were hurtling through the night at the speed of light, we were bound for some distant ranch, or a sweat lodge. That I would die, that was a fact. I had died before, many times, and now it was time to die again. Oh, the mystery, the pain, the wonder and the why of it all.

They say the sense of hearing is the last to go and the first to come back. When at last the fever broke and the coughing began, I woke to noise. Disembodied voices, the buzz and hum of medical equipment, the incessant beep, a nagging reminder that somewhere, someone's IV needed attention. I recognized the masked figures caring for me, not by name but by profession. Nurses, they knew what to do. A nurse had my back. The lone gunman was nowhere in sight, but if he came for me, if he had a bullet with my name on it, the nurse would listen like a priest, accept my shortcomings and grant me my last request. A nurse would ease my pain, brush my hair, bring my children to say goodbye.

This bug, you can't kill it with a bullet. The body can fight it but, in the end, it's up to the lone gunman whether I live or die. With any luck and a lot of science, there will be a vaccine, but sure as shootin' a new bug will come along. There is no place left to hide, not even in your dreams.

I am a child again, riding in the back seat of the buckboard half asleep or half awake, the vibration relaxing me, loosening my thoughts, jiggling them away from my brittle joints, freeing my soul. Cholera hit the wagon train, killed so many of us that year. Killed the natives too, like the smallpox and the diphtheria. Killed more than bullets, these bugs. Still, the nurse cared for me.

If I die, let it be a burning revelation, a cool drink of relief, a glorious reward. Death, the lone gunman, an afternoon nap, a morning dream, a morphine dream. I'm dreaming I'm playing poker at the big golden table and I'm there, standing in line to be born, waiting to be dealt my card, a luckier card this time.

Calamity

It had only been five days since she had last seen her mother in person, felt her strong hands comb the tangles from her hair, making her eyes sting, before parting it in a straight line on her scalp and making two braids down her back. She liked it when mommy fixed her hair, even though it hurt a little bit. Today, she had finally let Abuela brush and braid her hair, but it didn't feel quite the same when she did it. Even when mommy was at work, all night long, she knew she was helping people, that was her job. Now, the bug had got her mother and the other nurses were taking care of her. But she should be all better by now. Mommy was strong and Calamity wanted her.

"Wyatt, when is mommy coming home?"

Her brother's eyes never left the screen, his thumbs furiously working the controller, trying his best to stay alive, and to kill the last bad guy left standing. If he knew, he wasn't saying.

∞

'This is the beginning of the end of something.'

Katherine Anne Porter
Pale Horse, Pale Rider

A heartfelt thanks to the caregivers on the frontline and in the trenches of

healthcare delivery during the 2020 pandemic.

Nurse Kit Carson's Adventures

A series of short stories by L.S. Collison

available in electronic format, collectible paperbacks, and audio

Friday Night Knife & Gun Club
Saturday Night Knife & Gun Club
Sunday Night Knife & Gun Club
Monday Night Knife & Gun Club

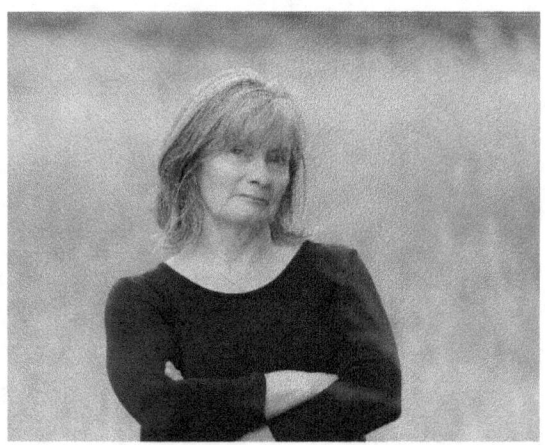

author photo - PhotoZ by Sheila. Sheila Zappanti
cover design by M.G. Manelis
editorial consultation by S.K. Keogh

www.fictionhouseltd.com

www.lindacollison.com